Submissive Training

The Uncensored and Shameless History and Facts Guide About BDSM

By: More Sex More Fun Book Club

Table of Contents

Introduction

I want to thank you and congratulate you for purchasing the book, *"**BDSM Playbook For Beginners.**"*

This book contains proven steps and strategies on how to explore the concept of BDSM to bring about amazing improvements in your sex life and in your relationship.

Imagine yourself and your partner playing a game. Your lover stands behind you while you lean backward, eyes closed, and you let yourself fall, trusting your lover to catch you. Certain thoughts will probably race through your mind.

Will your lover catch you?

Will he/she let you fall?

Will he/she be able to catch you in time?

And yet, despite the risks, when everything goes exactly as planned, the both of you experience an incomparably exhilarating sensation. *This is what BDSM is all about*: Trust. Excitement. An incomparable intimate experience.

Sadly, Mainstream movies and cheap erotica have tainted people's perception of BDSM. These days, a lot of people misconstrue BDSM as an abusive and bizarre practice. In fact, BDSM is about respect. It's not about striking fear. It's about conquering fear. BDSM is when trust, confidence, and curiosity win over the possibility of pain or harm or humiliation. Through this book, you will learn the true definition of BDSM, the origins and the basics, and more importantly, the benefits of introducing BDSM to your relationship.

During sex, you need to be involved not just physically but mentally and emotionally as well. BDSM makes you available and vulnerable to your partner in all three dimensions and vice versa, thus deepening your intimacy. Through these pages, you will discover the basic steps to incorporating BDSM into your sex life from proper communication to basic BDSM sex techniques to recommended tools and toys for beginners.

Thanks again for purchasing this book. I hope you enjoy it!

Chapter 1: BDSM Demystified

Nowadays, BDSM is often used to describe a broad range of erotic practices that are perceived as beyond ordinary, and even deviant. But if you've ever blindfolded your lover, if you've ever spanked your partner for naughty behavior, or if you've ever teased someone by briefly withholding sexual pleasure, then you've taken the baby steps to BDSM.

Contrary to what most people may believe, BDSM is far from being a modern sex fad. BDSM has been practiced for centuries though the acronym was first used between the 50's and the 60's.

- **B** stands for Bondage which refers to the use of restraints in order to heighten sexual pleasure.

- **D** stands for Discipline, which refers to the use of punishment and reward in order to control sexual behavior.

- **D&S** stands for Dominance and Submission which is commonly perceived as power play. D&S relationships need not necessarily be physical. In fact, there are a lot of Dom-Sub relationships online. Furthermore, Dom-Sub relationships aren't all that black and white. Couples may choose to switch roles from time to time. Meanwhile, some individuals have a tendency to develop a taste for the opposite role throughout the course of time.

- **S&M** means Sadism and Masochism which is usually where some people get their impression of BDSM. But as you are discovering now, there is more to BDSM than just whips and chains.

This acronym is that which ties together various sexual activities that may seem to have nothing in common at all.

Others use the term BDSM to describe a fetish. Others use it to describe a lifestyle.

BDSM is more than just spanking or playing the role of the sub or the dom. BDSM is a great many things. It's about taking control. It's about relinquishing control. It's about inflicting physical pain to show love and respect. It's about taking the pain to show love and respect. It's that human beast of burden pulling a cart. It's turning your sex partner into a foot stool. It's mild hair pulling. It's suspending your sexual soulmate from the ceiling. It's keeping your lover on his/her toes... figuratively and literally. It's donning costumes and assuming a role. It's cock worship. It's forced bedwetting. It's a kidnapping fantasy. It's a nipple-pinching, ball-crushing, butt-bruising game. BDSM can be all these things and more. Yet it can never be used to exclusively define a single fetish or activity.

More importantly, BDSM is a consensual act and an agreement made between two responsible individuals who want to bring their sexual experience to new heights. Ultimately, BDSM is a shared adventure where couples become free to explore their innermost fantasies, to discover their boundaries, and to push those boundaries.

BDSM is an exploration of the self. It is an exploration of one's partner. It is an exploration of one's willingness to be truthful to oneself and to one's partner. It is not a dehumanizing act. Rather, it is the most *human* form of lovemaking there is. Animals may have sex without talking, planning or negotiating but in BDSM sex, boundaries are made clear, setups are arranged, needs are addressed, and emotions are nurtured.

Chapter 2: The History of Kink

Records found by anthropologists dating back to 4000-3100 BCE in early Mesopotamia showed evidences of festivities and sacrifices which involve domination, cross-dressing, giving and taking of pain for pleasure, and altered states of consciousness.

Graphical proof of sadomasochism was discovered in an Estrucan burial site dating back to 6th Century BCE. It was a depiction of two men whipping one woman with the use of their bare hands and a cane while assuming an erotic position.

In the Kama Sutra (300 CE), you'll find sections which refer to sexual practices that involve pain and pleasure. According to the book, you must only inflict pain upon women who agree to receive it. Hence, the Kama Sutra provides us with the earliest record of consensual kinky sex.

There were references to BDSM activities in 15th century Europe though it became more public in the 18th century when brothels which specialized in flagellation, bondage, and "acts of punishment" began to flourish. During this time, dominant female prostitutes were available to meet the needs of submissive men.

In 1886, Richard Freiherr von Krafft-Ebing popularized the term Sadomasochism in his book *Psychopathia Sexualis*. Sigmund Freud utilized the word to describe a kind of neurotic sexual enjoyment. The term got its origins from the combined names of Marquis de Sade and Leopold von Sacher-Masoch. Both men were highly controversial authors during their time.

Marquis the Sade lived in France from 1740 to 1840. He bore the reputation of a worst libertine. He wrote several semi-fictional works which included heavily sexual scenes, something which the Catholic Church frowned upon. However, the philosopher and the aristocrat did more than just that. His stories and his plays depicted scenes that were not only regarded as erotic but also as violent and illegal. Take his work, "Juliette" as an example. It told the tale of an orphan girl who had just ripened to puberty. She was taken into a convent and there at the nunnery, she was initiated by the Mother Superior to acts of pleasure, from performing cunnilingus to using dildos. Other scenes in his works involved priests, nuns, and even the Pope kissing, fucking, masturbating with prostitutes and with each other, defecating and urinating on each other, and even hurting or killing each other violently while they're at it. Naturally, this infuriated the Catholic Church. The Marquis was locked up in an insane asylum for 32 years but that didn't stop him from writing and having his stories smuggled to be released to the public. The point is, the Marquis de Sade also practiced what he preached (or at least most of it) and for this, the term Sadism was created after his name.

The Austrian Leopold Ritter von Sacher-Masoch who was born many years later after the Marquis (1836) was known for his published work, *Venus in Furs* where he elaborated on the concept of the dominant female. In this book, the man falls in love with a woman, volunteers to be her slave, and begs her to treat him in a degrading manner. As time passes, the acts gradually become more and more degrading. Like de Sade, von Sacher-Masoch practiced what he preached and even asked his wife to play the role of the dom and to do unto him exactly what's written in the book. Thus, it was only appropriate that the term Masochism was taken from his name.

It was in 1950's when Irving Klaw's black and white photos and films came out featuring the gorgeous pin-up model Bettie Page. Sometimes, she was bound and gagged, playing the role of the sub. Sometimes, she held the whip in her hands, playing the role of the dom.

Nowadays, the internet provides readers with all sorts of misleading info about BDSM causing them to get turned off

Chapter 3: Better than Vanilla: Benefits of BDSM

BDSM leads to better sex

Great sex is when you can be free to be yourself with your lover -- no hang-ups, no pretenses. This is what you get with BDSM sex. Imagine how liberating it is to know that you're having sex with the *real* version of your partner.

Great sex requires variety and couples who practice BDSM are constantly expending time and effort in finding ways to make sex more exciting for each other. Trying one sexual adventure after the other enhances your curiosity and your confidence in bed.

Great sex is a result of great foreplay. Often in BDSM sex, there is constant touching involved. It's not the mindless, mechanical coupling that usually occurs during vanilla sex. In order for BDSM sex to work, it requires you to be aware, to be in the present, to be an active participant. And isn't that what a healthy relationship is all about?

BDSM leads to better communication in relationships

In order to have great sex, it's important that you don't just *do* it. You also need to be able to *talk* about it. Keeping all of your needs and fantasies to yourselves inevitably leads to dissatisfaction, frustration, and resentment towards each other. Couples who engage in BDSM are more communicative when it comes to expressing their sexual desires. In turn, they also become more open in expressing their deepest emotions.

In vanilla relationships, couples don't usually talk openly about sex. They don't confront their partner's shortcomings or wonder about their own until such a time when their relationship or marriage becomes threatened. BDSM couples, before they even bother exploring this lifestyle. This is something that we are going to correct through this book.

on the other hand, are naturally honest and direct with each other because they need transparency in order for the BDSM relationship to thrive. In fact, most BDSM couples tend to develop a secret language that only the two of them can understand. Each time you talk about rules and safe words or make a list of things that you want to do between the sheets, you are actively communicating and considering each other's needs.

BDSM increases intimacy between couples

When couples do something new together, this makes them vulnerable to each other. When you share an adventure with each other, the experience binds you. How can it not? You share a secret together. You've shared one euphoric moment after the next. Moreover, that feeling of bliss that you experience each time you try something new is automatically linked to your partner. Thus, when you think of each other, you end up feeling the exciting sensation all over.

This goes without saying but each time you let your lover bind you, or blindfold you, or flog you, it necessitates a high degree of trust which is essential in all relationships.

BDSM promotes fidelity

Contrary to what most people may believe, BDSM relationships do not often lead to lewd sexual behavior, multiple sexual partners, and infidelity. In fact, couples who take BDSM seriously end up investing a great deal of time, energy, trust, and emotion into the relationship that it would be less likely for them to do anything to sabotage their efforts. They are unlikely to risk all the trust and safety that they have painstakingly built. Furthermore, two of the major causes of infidelity are sexual incompatibility and stagnation. Both rarely apply in BDSM relationships.

BDSM aids in improving mental health

Studies reveal that BDSM friendly individuals are less fearful, more open-minded, more secure in relationships, and better at coping with rejection. According to research, BDSM has therapeutic effects to individuals who have experienced psychological trauma in the past. That's because it allows you to express your sexuality without fear or shame. BDSM sex requires you and your partner to be fully present: mind, body, and soul during the interaction and thus the therapeutic powers of BDSM can be likened to that of yoga or mindful meditation.

BDSM lessens psychological stress and anxiety

A scientific experiment revealed that while participating in BDSM activities, the subjects' stress levels have noticeably decreased. Both dominants and submissives reflected lower cortisol levels in their systems. That's because in BDSM sex, you let go of expectations and judgment to give way to physical intensity. While observing both sub and dom subjects engage in giving and taking pain, scientists discovered decreased blood flow in the prefrontal and limbic pain regions in the brain. This yields a tranquilizing effect, thus lessening anxiety.

BDSM encourages self-advocacy

Who you are in bed is a reflection of who you are in real life. If you're frightened, anxious, or uptight between the sheets, that's who you are at home and at work. Whether or not it is manifested externally, it's who you are inside.

Participating in BDSM sex helps you become more honest and more upfront about your sexual needs. When you learn to confidently speak out in the bedroom by giving a command, that's when you stop being a person who just sits and wait for others to anticipate your needs. When you learn to speak a safe word during BDSM sex, that's when you stop becoming that person who's too afraid to interrupt someone mid-speech regardless of how uncomfortable you're feeling.

BDSM teaches responsibility

Whether you are a sub or a dom, BDSM teaches you that you are responsible for the quality of your sexual experience. Being a dominant is not about taking advantage of your power to suit only your selfish desires just as being a submissive is not about shutting your brain off so you could let your partner do all the work. BDSM is all about establishing a give-and-take relationship.

Some people mistake the role of the submissive as a powerless position and thus, one that is free from any responsibility. On the contrary, there is a special kind of power that the submissive possesses over the dominant. It's the sub who decides how long he/she will continue to give away his/her control. The moment the sub uses the safe word, the dom must stop. Once the submissive decides that he/she will no longer relinquish power, the Sub-Dom relationship is over.

Chapter 4: The Basics of BDSM

It all begins with the self

The first step would be to educate yourself. Learn to differentiate between fantasy and desire. Erotic fantasies reside in your imagination and as such, they have no limits. Desires, on the other hand, is something which you crave for in reality. So while you may allow your fantasy to go crazy, you have to be realistic about what you truly desire for your relationship and your sex life.

Naturally, you'll need to be honest with yourself about whether you're more of a sub or more of a dom. If you're a sub, what kind of sub are you, specifically? Are you a babygirl/mommy's little boy? Or are you more of a slave? There are so many levels to submission just as there are so many levels to domination.

But more than that, you need to be specific about the kind of erotic energy you want to try out. A touch can be nurturing, teasing, cruel, or agonizing, all depending on the erotic energy which you place behind it. For instance, you can't just ask your partner to spank you. It doesn't work like that. You need to be crystal clear about the kind of spanking that you desire. Do you want it to be light and playful? Heavy and rough? You need to reflect on all these things or else you'll end up not getting exactly what you want.

It's also important to ask yourself what BDSM means to you because this will determine where you must begin. Are you more interested in the B&D part or in the S&M part? If you're more into B&D, then it's recommended that you start off with simple blindfolding. If you're more into S&M, then it's best to start off with some mild spanking.

Basic BDSM Roles: *Subs... Doms... Which is which?*

- **Mistress** or **Domme** is a term used to describe the female dominant. She controls the pace of the sex and must be obeyed.

- The **Master** is the male dominant.

- The **Daddy** is a kind of male dominant where the submissive is called the **Babygirl.** Though possessing a dominant role, he is more nurturing compared to the Master.

- The female version of the Daddy is called the **Mommy**.

- It is important to note that the **Babygirl** or the **Daddy's Little Girl** is not an underage girl. She is, in fact, a grown woman who enjoys being in contact with her inner child. The male counterpart is the **Mommy's Little Boy**.

- The **Brat** is a kind of babygirl who acts out in a rebellious, child-like manner so as to provoke the Dominant to spank him/her.

- The **Submissive** refers to the individual who relinquishes power to the Dominant. Note that being a submissive doesn't necessarily mean that one is weak or clingy. In fact, people who possess power roles in their careers like bosses of great companies enjoy fulfilling the role of the submissive because it provides them with a welcome respite from having to make all the decisions. It gives them a brief moment to be carefree.

- Compared to the Submissive, the **Slave** offers a more complete servitude to the Master or the Mistress with a desire to be fully owned and to be controlled by him/her. As such, a symbolic contract is often drawn. Thus, the role is performed not just during sex but outside the bedroom as well.

- The **Switch** is what you call an individual who likes being the dom but also likes being the sub. This also refers to couples who enjoy power exchange and swapping roles.

- The **Sadist** is someone who takes pleasure in giving either physical or emotional pain or humiliation. Meanwhile, the **Masochist** is someone who takes pleasure in receiving it. Remember that all pain inflicted and all humiliations are consensual. Note that just because someone is the Dom, it doesn't mean that he's the Sadist in the relationship. He can, in fact, be the one giving the command but also the one receiving the pain. Hence, it's not necessary to be a sadist to be a dom and vice versa. A **Sadomasochist** is someone who enjoys receiving pain just as much as he enjoys giving it.

Have the Talk

There is no other way to go about it but to sit together and have an honest and mature conversation with each other. Start off by sharing your deepest, most secret desires with each other. Create an erotic bucket list, if you must. Listen to your partner's desires and encourage him/her to be honest by being honest yourself.

There are several ways in which you can prepare your significant other for the talk. For instance, you can read to him/her an erotic scene from a book that you love then ask your partner what he/she thinks about it.

E.g.: "That scene in "Secretary" where Maggie Gyllenhaal got spanked by her boss for her typos was pretty hot wasn't it?"

Explain to your partner what intrigued you most about that scene. You can say something like this:

"What fascinated me was how powerful the guy must've felt when he forced her to read through her typos while spanking her bum raw. He must've felt like he was helping her learn a lesson she'll never forget. I loved how she enjoyed it too... being obedient, having her mistakes corrected without feeling offended."

You can even venture so far as to say something like:

"How would feel like if I do that to you every time you say a swear word?"

Whatever your lover's reaction is, take in a non-judgmental manner.

Here's another more straightforward approach:

"I had a dream where one of us was in charge during lovemaking. What do you think about that?"

When talking about your individual fantasies, the rule is to never say never. Have an open mind and don't automatically dismiss your partner's suggestions. If you think that your significant other's desires are a little too kinky for you, negotiate. Instead of saying: "No, I won't." or "No, I can't.", say: "Maybe not now." Or "We'll see."

If your partner is worried or anxious about incorporating BDSM into your sexual activities, discuss it without putting any pressure on him/her. Explore what his/her fears are. What is he/she worried about? What are the factors that have caused this negative idea of BDSM?

Don't believe everything that you see on the internet. Remind your partner that he/she doesn't have to do anything that they don't want to. In the end, BDSM sex is what you make it.

Set boundaries

Once you and your partner have both agreed to engage in BDSM sex, it's time to set the ground rules.

This is where you take into consideration your individual comfort zones. A checklist may be made just to be sure that you really are on the same page.

For example, if you're planning to explore bondage, discuss exactly how you're willing to be bound. Are you okay with your hands and feet being tied? Or would you be more comfortable if only your hands were tied and your legs are left free? When you're all tied up, what are the things that your partner are allowed to do? You may be okay with your partner kissing and touching you while you're all tied up but you may not be okay with sexual penetration while you're still bound. You need to be very specific.

Here are some examples of setting boundaries:

"Yes, you can put ice on my clitoris but never insert it into my vagina. Also, I'm uncomfortable doing this while I'm blindfolded and tied up."

"Yes, I'm okay with sex toys being inserted into my anus but dildos have to be four inches or shorter. I'm not sure if I'm ready for vibrating toys. I'm not comfortable with having anything attached to my penis."

"I loved being spanked anywhere except on the face."

The Negotiation phase is where you identify the roles that you're going to play. Are you top or bottom? Are you sub or dom?

This is also where you come up with the Safeword which will be used if either of you feels uncomfortable. Be sure that the safeword is something that the both of you will easily remember and that it's not something that you would normally say during sex.

For example, don't use "No", "Stop.", or "Please, don't." as a safeword as it can easily be misconstrued as part of one's roleplaying. Instead, say something like: "Candy." or "Clover". You should also prepare for cases where safewords may not be used, like when the sub's mouth is gagged or when you're playing music loudly; for such cases, create the applicable safe signal. It can be a hand gesture (or a head gesture if the hands are tied).

Some couples create two different safewords where one means "slow down" while the other means "stop now".

Once you have established your rules, stick to them. Even when, at the heat of the moment, you become tempted to take things one step farther, or even if you see that your partner can take some harder spanking, fight the urge and stick to the rules. It's way better to leave your partner wanting more than to turn him/her off from BDSM forever. You can always renegotiate afterwards.

Take it one step at a time.

Always start with the feather before moving on to the whip. The greatest mistake that couples make is trying out too many things at one time. Another is immediately trying out toys and positions that are too complicated.

So before you start tying your partner's wrists to the bed, try pining her arms up with your hands and see how she feels about this. Before inserting dildos into your guy's anus, why not start first with a gloved and well-lubricated finger and see if he's really comfortable with it. Explore one element at a time. Don't start off by combining bondage and whips in one go.

The key is to gradually build up the intensity. Have your partner rate your spanking from a scale of one to ten (ten being the hardest that your lover can take, NOT the hardest that you can give).

Evaluate constantly

It is necessary to communicate after sharing a BDSM experience. Talk to each other to find out whether expectations have been met and how you can improve the experience for the next session. Are you willing to take it to the next level? Should you take it down a notch? Or should you stay where you are at the moment?

Remember: Always Secure Consent

One great rule in BDSM sex is to "Never Assume Anything." Consent is important because it's the fine line which distinguishes kinky sex from abuse. It doesn't matter if you've been having BDSM sex for years. Consent is crucial. Consent is a solid "Yes" from your partner. This means that he/she understands the consequences of the activity because you've discussed it beforehand. This is how men and women feel safe when assuming the role of the submissive. They are not fearful about what's going to happen next because they already know what to expect. Thus, they are free to relinquish control to their partners. Likewise, this is how dominants feel safe about assuming their roles. It's how they know that whatever it is that they do, it is wanted, welcomed, and enjoyed by their partner.

Before engaging in any form of BDSM activity, ask your partner plainly: "Before we begin, I must know that you've agreed to this."

Chapter 5: BDSM Tools and Toys for Beginners

BDSM is a fantasy. In fact, think of it as a play that requires a plot, a setting, costumes, and tools.

Not everyone can afford to have his/her own red room of pain but with a few tweaks, you can magically transform your boudoir anytime into a shrine of pleasure. Turn your bedroom into a sacred space exclusive for sleeping and lovemaking. More importantly, turn it into a judgment-free zone.

Make use of aromatherapy candles and oils and install dim lighting to help set the mood. If you're planning on making BDSM love during the daytime, invest in thick curtains and blinds. You're going to be indulging in a fantasy so get rid of stuff that will distract you and remind you of your personal life. (ex. the laundry list that screams "plain housewife" instead of "Domme" or that mobile phone which will remind you that you're not "Mommy's little boy."

BDSM tools don't necessarily need to be physical. In fact, at the beginning, you're advised to start with simple tools which can be found at home. The real turn on in BDSM is the *idea* of dominating or being dominated. Thus, it's something that you can do with or without the use handcuffs or whips.

You can start assuming the dominant role by ordering your lover to lie supine on the bed.

Tell him/her exactly where to place his/her arms. Do this with utmost confidence. Your voice, your expression, your body langue speaks louder than the whip in your hand.

Ultimately, the most important thing in BDSM sex is to weave a spell and to believe in that fantasy.

Before purchasing BDSM tools reminiscent of the Spanish Inquisition, why not look around your home for tamer toys.

You can also blindfold the sub with an eye mask. Bind him/her with a silk tie before progressing to handcuffs. Then use a clean feather duster to tickle your partner with. As mentioned, as a beginner, it would be more fun not to jump straight to using sex toys. Instead, use your imagination to utilize torture tools which are available to you. Your tongue! Lick your partner's body in random places while withholding pleasure.

Go easy and don't fast-forward to using ball gags for the mouth. Experiment with a suit tie first.

For spanking, start off by using the back of a hairbrush or a spatula instead of a whip.

If you want to explore animal play, don't begin by wrapping a dog collar around your partner's neck. Start off by wrapping a small collar around the wrist or the arm then lead him/her around the room or house.

Do you think that you're ready for bloodsports (pricking the skin for pain and to draw small amounts of blood)? Well don't go there just yet! Start off by using a tracing wheel. Roll it around your partner's sensitive parts (ex. around the nipples, near the groin) and see if they're comfortable with it.

Before using nipple clamps, test the waters by pinching your partner's nipples.

If you're into S&M, another household tool you can use is a candle. Start with one or two drops of hot wax into your partner's least sensitive body part.

BDSM Toys for the Big Boys (and Girls)

Floggers

The trick in choosing floggers is to determine exactly what kind of stimulation you're after. This will depend entirely on the thongs' width and the material they're made of. When purchasing leather floggers, a softer type of leather is more advisable for beginners. In fact, it's recommended to opt for the suede variety which will provide a milder sting and can help warm up your skin. Thin thongs made from rubber or stiff ones made from tough leather can inflict more pain especially when the whips are administered with force.

Crops

If you're ready for them, you can purchase crops from riding stores. Remember though that the stiffer the crop is, the greater the sting. Also, the smaller the tip/tongue is, the more it is capable to inflict pain.

Canes

The thinner canes are, the more they are likely to hurt and even break the submissive's skin. Soft blows with thicker canes are more recommended for newbies *after* some practice with the hairbrush or the spatula. One technique is to not actually hit the submissive but to tease him/her by blindfolding him/her and then swishing the cane in the air rapidly and really hard.

Nipple Clamps

Beginners are better off with the screw-up variety which can be adjusted. The technique is to start off by leaving the nipple clamps on the sub's nips for a maximum of two minutes. The moment you remove the clamps, that's the time when the sub will actually feel the pain as the blood comes rushing back to that area.

Paddles

The rule for choosing paddles is that the wider and stiffer it is, the more intense the pain will be. Opt for soft suede paddles. Naturally, you should start off with flat paddles before experimenting with studded ones.

Restraints

In choosing restraints, opt for ones that have broad straps that fit well. They are recommended to ensure comfort during lengthy roleplaying scenes.

If you plan on using ropes then be sure that they don't put pressure on any tendons or ligaments. It would be extremely uncomfortable for the submissive if there's an enormous knot pressing against his/her back as he/she is lying down.

Once you and your partner decide that you're ready for neck collars, remember this rule: Never leave the sub unattended if his/her neck collar is attached to any object.

Your Imagination

Your brain is undoubtedly the most valuable BDSM tool there is. Unlike any sex toy, your imagination possesses unrivaled potential in building excitement and fantasy.

One thing you can do is to send erotic text messages or emails to each other during the day. Tease your lover and build the passion to a crescendo by telling your sexual soulmate exactly what you plan to do to him/her.

As mentioned, Sub-Dom relationships often occur online without any physical contact.

For example, a Dom can easily call his/her Submissive and order him/her exactly what to eat for dinner. "I want you to eat three slices of carrots, one pea, and a matchbox sized chicken meat. No skin. Now, take three small sips of wine."

Don't underestimate the power of language. Use personal honorifics to refer to your sub/dom. You can call your sub your "kitten", or your dom your "Queen."

In the end, remember that BDSM sex is a deeply personalized experience. It is only as wild or as dangerous or as exciting as you make it. As mentioned earlier, BDSM is such a broad term that can mean a lot of things but ultimately, it is what you make it to be, from a fun one-night thing to a rich lifetime experience.

Chapter 6: Social Aspects to BDSM

Believe it or not, the BDSM community is just that, a community! There are rules that are going to have to be put in place to respect both parties and ensure that they are being safe. But, there are other parts to the community than just that.

Top or bottom?

There are two roles when it comes to BDSM. The top and the bottom. When you look at the two roles, you can put them on a scale of one to ten. At the low end, there is someone who is going to be able to reject any physical stimulation while at the other end are those who are knows as the bottoms. Bottoms highly enjoy humiliation and discipline because they are not wanting to be submissive to the person who is giving it out. Thus, they are usually the person who sets the conditions for the session that they are going to participate in and will dole out the instructions in the negotiation process.

Tops are going to respect guidance and not act out as often because they do not want to be disciplined. Some bottoms are known to be called brats because they purposely misbehave so that they can be punished. However, topping from the bottom is considered to be rude inside the standards of most traditional BDSM relationships.

Relationship types

Just like you are used to seeing different types of relationships in the "real" world, in the BDSM world, there are different types of relationships as well.

Play

For some, BDSM is only a part of their sex life and it is consistent of roleplaying or "playing". Play will be inside of a session and there are constraints put on the session or scene.

Sometimes this sort of relationship involves kink play or other BDSM activities.

Long term

There was not much written on long term relationships in BDSM until recently. In 2003, there was a study to look into long term relationships that were between those who practiced the lifestyle. Those who participated in the study said that their BDSM orientation was part of who they were and they did not choose it. However, many of them were able to compromise and match what their partner's needs were.
Most found that the perfect partner was the one that had the same interest that they did, but, like any relationship certain wants and desires aside to keep the relationship going. Some of the activities that these couples partook in were both sexual and nonsexual in nature. It was reported that when a couple participated in BDSM bonded more and released stress. One thing though was that the roles of submissive and dominant were kept through the entire day because it was too hard to switch back and forth.

In the same study, the ones who identified as a bottom were the ones who played harder and had more constrictions on their role whenever what they wanted did not match what their partner wanted. The author of the study made the prediction that those who thought themselves to be tops were not in the mood to play as often since there was an increased demand on them to make sure that both parties were safe.

It was stated by the author of the study that long term BDSM relationships were established early and there had to be full disclosure from both parties in what was to come from the relationship.

People participating in long term BDSM relationships tend to learn from others in the BDSM community. Many believe that the top is the one who were holding the most control when it came to the relationship. But, there are no beliefs that the top being better than the bottom in any fashion.

In the study, it was written: "The respondents valued themselves, their partners, and their relationships. All couples expressed considerable good will towards their partners. The power exchange between the cohorts appears to be serving purposes beyond any sexual satisfaction, including experiencing a sense of being taken care of and bonding with a partner."

As the study continued, three different aspects were discussed in how a long term BDSM relationship works. The full disclosure of interests, using their roles in the relationship as a tool to keep the relationship, and a commitment for personal growth. Because of how serious the threat for harm was in these relationships, communication was higher than most other relationships so that both parties were kept safe.

Professional services

Professional services are for those who offer all of the BDSM services in exchange for an agreed upon price. You will find professional dominants and dominatrix, but a dominatrix is less talked about. A woman who is not a professional dominant is known as a domme or femdom.

You can also purchase a female submissive that will do as is asked of her but inside the terms of a negotiated contract and most only work inside of professional dungeons so that there are people there in case something goes wrong. A professional submissive is going to be a little harder to locate, but they are out there.

Those that offer up their submissive services tend to enjoy sadomasochism.

Males that identify as a top are the masters and can be harder to find. A pro-dom male is normally going to only work with males.

Scenes

Scenes are going to be staged and BDSM activity is going to take place. Normally the scene takes place in a dungeon where it is a controlled location and both people are taken care of. Many people do not like the term dungeon and therefore they call it a play space. Not all play that happens in a scene involves sexual activity.

For many relationships that involve BDSM, the main characteristic is the power exchange that happens whenever a dominant partner takes control of the submissive partner through bondage and other sexual roleplay.

Scene does not just refer to the roleplay that partners participate in, it also involves the entire BDSM community. If you are on the "scene" then you are wanting to play in a public setting and you may even participate in play at a public party.
Scenes typically take place between two or more people and can include anything from master and slave relationships to servitude. There are BDSM elements that are going to be included that include punishment during slave training whenever instructions are not followed as they are supposed to be.

A few people enjoy being watched by others so their scenes take place in BDSM clubs and the equipment that is used is made available for use while having others there to watch ensures that there is safety for those in the scene, especially if the partners are strangers.

Etiquette

Just because it is a different type of community does not mean that there are not rules.

- Do not touch a person that you do not know

- Do not touch what belongs to someone else which includes their toys.

- Follow the dress code

Even if the event is open to the public, there are going to be rules that have to be followed. These rules are going to address things such as drugs, alcohol, photography, and cell phones.

There are even rules inside of a scene which include things like making sure that both parties are comfortable with what is going on and consent to the entire scene before it even starts. All clubs are going to have rules on how an onlooker may interact with the scene if it is permitted by the players.

Parties and clubs

There are events that are going to be held by those who participate in BDSM are for those who are interested and gives them the opportunity to share their experiences and knowledge. There is also the opportunity to play in a setting where it is accepted by everyone that is there. These parties are going to have a strict dress code and most of what you see people in attendance wearing is leather, latex, or anything else that will show off their bodies.

Acts of BDSM are performed publicly or privately depending on the party and those participating. When play is done in a dungeon, toys that are not typically available in homes are available such as a spanking bench or other large equipment. Plus, you do not have to worry about the noise that comes from using such equipment.

Most BDSM parties allow for exhabtionists as well as voyeurs to participate in an environment free of judgement. However, intercourse is not allowed at such parties since it is not what

BDSM play is about. It is also a matter of safety and comfort for the players so that others are not seeing what may be an intimate part of their relationship. You can find BDSM parties in larger cities in the Western world.

One of the largest BDSM events you will find is the Folsom Street Fair. A few others are:

- Living in Leather

- Black rose

- Shibaricon

- Spankfest

Chapter 7: The Psychology Behind BDSM

One of the most common misconceptions behind BDSM is that it comes from being abused as a child. However, there is no research that supports this claim. There are a few reports that indicate that a child that was abused is going to have more injuries while participating in BDSM activities and are not going to be able to say their safe word because they feel like they deserve what is being done to them. There is also another link that shows those of the transgender that are abused are going to be abused when they are participating in BDSM.

Studies have shown that there are a lot of reasons that a person wants to participate in a sadomasochist relationship and finds that S&M is enjoyable to them. But, each answer is going to only come from the individual because everyone gets into BDSM for a different reason. There are a few that find taking on the role of the submissive and not having a say in what happens is an escape from everything that goes on in their everyday life. Others still think that they are going to find safety and protection that they did not find in their childhood or they are seeking approval from an authoritarian figure that they did not get as a child.

Someone who enjoys being a sadist could enjoy having all of the power thus are going to be the ones who take on a more dominant role and receive their pleasure through what they do to the masochist. No one actually understands what connects the emotions that they are feeling to the sexual gratification that they are getting.

Psychiatry adviser Joseph Merlino said in an interview: "It's not a problem only if it is getting that individual into difficulties, if he or she is nto happy with it, or it's causing problems in their personal or professional lives. If it's not, I'm not seeing that as a problem. But assuming that it did, what I would wonder about is what his or her biology that would cause a tendency towar a problem, and dynamically, what were the experiences this individual had that led him or her toward one of the ends of the spectrum."

There are many other psychologist that say that one's experience early on as they were developing sexually, is going to have a profound effect on that person later on in their sexuality. The desires for sadomasochistic can be formed at any age. There are reports of a few people having these feelings before they eve hit puberty and yet others have found that they enjoy BDSM later on when they were adults.

There is a study that says about fifty three percent of the males that enjoy sadomasochist found that they enjoy this before they were even fifteen while about seventy eight percent of females showed their interest after the age of fifteen. There are less female sadists than male, however, the sadistic fantasies occur in both men and women.

In a study of those who took part in masochistic sessions found the behavior to be addictive giving off some of the same effects that one may experience if they were taking drugs.

Prevalence

BDSM is practiced by both homo and hetrosexual men and women on many different levels. There are some couples that had absolutely nothing to do with the BDSM culture outside of their bedroom all the way to those who take part in public events.

In 1953 it was stated that about twelve percent of females and twenty two percent of males experience some sort of response when they hear about what goes on in a BDSM scene.

There have been many other studies that show numbers just appear to go up when it comesto showing interest in BDSM as well as those what participated in some kind of BDSM activity such as using ties or blindfolds in the bedroom.

Recent studies

Back in 2014 there was a study done that involved college students from Canada as well as some people online. There were both males and females that participated in this study and it was found that nineteen percent of the males and ten percent of the females were able to find the sadistic scenarios that they read about as arousing to them in some fashion.

Out of some medical students that were interviewed the results that were found out were quite interesting.

Those that had been restrained:

- Straight men: twelve percent

- Gay men: twenty percent

- Bisexual men: thirteen percent

- Straight women: nineteen percent

- Gay women: thirty eight percent

- Bisexual women: fifty five percent.

Those that had restrained someone else for pleasure:

- Straight men: seventeen point five percent

- Gay men: seventeen percent

- Bisexual men: thirteen percent

- Straight women: thirteen percent

- Gay women: thirty six percent

- Bisexual women: fifty one percent

Had pain inflected upon them for pleasure:

- Straight men: four percent

- Gay men: six point five percent

- Bisexual men: eighteen percent

- Straight women: eight percent

- Gay women: ten percent

- Bisexual women: thirty six percent

Inflicted pain upon someone else for pleasure:

- Straight men: five percent

- Gay men: six percent

- Bisexual men: nine percent

- Straight women: four percent

- Gay women: six point five percent

- Bisexual women: twenty six percent

Medical

If you look at the most current version of the manual put out by the American Psychiatric Association, you will notice that BDSM is not one of the diagnosis for when someone experiences harm during sex. However, the International Classification of Diseases states that when you participate in mild forms of sadomasochistic activities, they can enhance what may be considered sexual activities that are normal. Many people participate in these taboo activities because of the stimulation and they find the sexual gratification they are looking for.

Sadomasochism was removed from the ICD in Europe thus making them the first European union to have it removed completely. Due to their movement, several other countries did the same thing being that those in the population who practiced BDSM were not harmed.

As of 2016, the ICD stated that as long as it is consensual there is nothing distressing or pathological against people participating in BDSM activities.

Coming out

There are some people who feel like they should come out in their sexual activities while a great majority do not tell anyone about their preferences. Anywhere from five all the way up to twenty five percent of the population show a fondness to the culture. There are even well known authors and other celebrities that are known as sadomasochist.

When it comes to female's there are two "camps" when discussing BDSM. Those that see it as a reflection of oppression and those who are pro-BDSM. However, some females have even criticized BDSM for making it okay to promote violence and power to males and those females that participate in BDSM are making women look bad.

Those females that are for BDSM on the other hand state that as long as the activities are consensual that it is validating the sexual inclinations for women and there is no actual link between participating in activities that are considered kinky and the sex crimes that are committed. Along with that, they should not attack how other women decide to show their sexual desires. It has been pointed out that the entire point behind feminism is to allow a woman free choices in her life and that is going to include how she chooses to express her sexual desires.

The roles that happen in BDSM are not fixed to one specific gender. Men can be submissive and females can be the dominant one. It also does not mean that men cannot have the same relationship with another man and two women cannot have the same relationship. In many relationships male/female, male/male, or female/ female, they switch roles depending on the situation that they are placed in.

Some studies have been done to see if there is a connection between BDSM pornography and violence that happens against women, and there has not been any connection found. If you take a look at Japan, you will come to realize that there are not many sexual crimes committed because of the industrialized nations that allow for BDSM and bondage pornography.

In '91, there was a survey that came to the conclusion between the years of 64 and 84 there was an increase in the sadomasochistic pornography that was available in the countries of Germany, Denmark, the United States, and Sweden. However, despite this, there is no link to the number of rape that is committed in that nation.

There was an operation done in the UK that was to prove that BDSM practitioners run a lower risk of being criminals just because of their sexual preferences. Around 2003, there was media coverage done on how participating and even working with a support group for BDSM added some risk to a person's job even when it came to a country that had no laws against BDSM. With some individuals, there is a strain that comes psychologically despite the fact that others know about them enjoying BDSM activities or not. It can however lead to a psychological situation that is going to be difficult because the person is going to be exposed to a high amount of emotional stress.

At the point in time that a person becomes aware of their desires towards BDSM scenarios and becomes open to it, this is called an internal coming out. In two different surveys, it was found that the amount of people who discovered this before their nineteenth birth increased. Sometimes people come out during an emotional crisis in their lives which can sometimes lead them to taking their own life, or thinking about it. This is why there have been support networks created in the past decades so that people have someone to go to when they are feeling like it is not going to work out for them and it does not go to where they feel they have no one to connect to.

Chapter 8: Cultural Aspects of BDSM

In most western countries, you can find people who participate in BDSM. This allows for those who participate others to talk to because they are likeminded and not going to judge. This is because BDSM is still considered to be unusual amongst the general public and they do not want others knowing that they are trying to learn about this subculture because it may make them appear as if they are weird.

Symbols

There are several different symbols that are going to indicate that someone is in the BDSM community. One of the most used symbols is the triskelion which is a circle. The triskele is used in various other cultures, however in the BDSM world it is from the Ring of O. The Emblem project has put a copyright on a specific version of the triskelion while other variations are free for claiming.

There is also a flag that is made especially for leather pride and it is widely used inside of the BDSM community.

Triskelion is going to be easy to see because it has three different pars that all stand for the BDSM acronym. While all three parts are separate, they are all connected and are normally associated together.

The rights flag is mean to show those that are in a relationship that leans towards BDSM and is meant to show that they believe that everyone, even though they practice BDSM deserves the same rights as others thus making it to where they should not be discriminated against just because they like something that is taboo.

The BDSM rights flag was originally inspired by the leather pride flag as well as the triskelion however it is mean to represent the fact that those who participate in BDSM have the same rights and it is not allowed to be used commercially.

Theatre

BDSM in theatre did not come around until contemporary theatre and because of that there are some plays that make it to where BDSM is the main theme of the play. There is one play that can be found in Austria and another in Germany that use BDSM as the main part of the play.

- Worauf sich Korper kaprizieren which is from Austria was wrote as a comedy and was later made into a film in the 50's. This play is about a marriage where the wife forces her husband and butler to submit to her so that she can find sexual gratification from her sadistic treatment. This goes on until two new characters take their place.

- Ache, Hilde (Oh, Hilda) is the German play where a young woman named Hilde becomes pregnant and then is abandoned by her boyfriend. In order to support herself and her child, she becomes a dominatrix so that she can earn the money that she needs.

Literature

Just like in theatre, you can find some of the literature that caters to BDSM and other fetish tastes that were created inside of early periods. But, you cannot find any BDSM literature that is earlier than World War II.

You can find the word sadism originating from Donatien Alphonse Francois, Marquis de Sade while the word masochism is from Leopold von Sacher-Masoch. Sadly, Marquis de Sade tended to write about abuse that was not mutual between the two parties. However, in his book *Venus in Furs* focused on a domme and sub relationship that was mutual between both parties.

One of the most notable works for BDSM is the *Story of O*.

The more recent work of E.L. James known as Fifty Shades has received a lot of criticism being that it was not accurate about how BDSM truly works between two partners despite how popular it became and still is.

Not all works of literature that involve BDSM are going to be accurate, however, there are some very accurate ones that you can find and those are the ones that you are going to want to stick to. There is nothing wrong with liking an erotic novel such as Fifty Shades, however, it should not be taken as how a true BDSM relationship works.

Art

- Photography: there are several well-known photographers that have taken pictures of bondage that is shown as erotic and sensual at the same time. Some of these works of art can be found in art museums, galleries and even private collections. One of the largest is known as the Baroness Marion Lambert's collection. There was a photographer in the late sixties and even early seventies that took pictures of BDSM and the homoeroticism that was part of his work was what pushed a national debate over the decision to give public funding to artwork or not should it be controversial.

- A Romanian songwriter got her musiv video banned in Romania because of the BDSM content for one of her songs known as Picture Perfect which was released in 2014.

- There are plenty of comic books that show BDSM of their heroines when they are captured by the bad guy, the same with graphic designs.

- Finally, there is a sculpture that is known as "The riding Crop" that shows a dominatrix that is wearing almost nothing using a riding crop one what one would assume to be her submissive.

Chapter 9: Pleasure Spots

Pleasure spots are not all about BDSM. Some of pleasure spots can be used when you are with your partner in a scene and being more intimate because being public with your relationship and private are two different things. Not to mention, pleasure spots are a great way to "torture" your partner!

Pleasure spots for her:

The first erogenous zone probably does not need much of an introduction, nor do we need to go into great detail on how to stimulate it. The **clitoris** is the zone with the most sexual arousal and sensitive nerves. Stimulating this zone is the fastest way to get a woman going. There are lots of ways to stimulate the clitoris. Rubbing gently with the pad of your thumb, vibrations, or licking with the flattest part of your tongue are all sure fire ways to make your lady moan. While your lady is on top, you can also press your thumb against her clit and rub in circles with a tempo matching her movements. Just know that simply touching the clitoris is not going to do much. The right amount of pressure or vibrations are what will work best.

The next zone is the **vagina.** In this zone, the walls of the vagina have tons of nerve endings. The inside reacts better to deeper penetration while the outside responds more positively to light touch or licking. Try teasing her by rubbing your fingers lightly across the lips of her sweet spot. You can also blow gently on it in between some light licking and sucking.

The **mouth and lips** are erogenous zones for women. Kissing is a great way to stimulate these areas and they are a direct line of energy to a woman's core. There are many ways to stimulate this part of the body. Taking the lower lip into your mouth and sucking gently, a little nip on that bottom lip is also a great move. Deep, passionate and even aggressive kisses are wonderful as well.

As it is with men, the **neck** is an erogenous zone for women. The nape of the neck is a great place to place soft kisses, give a little blow or flick of the tongue. Just under the jawline and underneath the earlobe are also really great places to land a few of those kisses. Go slow and tease her a bit.

Another couple of body parts that need no introduction and are probably obvious erogenous zones are the **breasts and nipples.** Like most erogenous zones on a woman's body, they are not one size fits all nor is there one particular place that will always be a turn on for women. The breasts are in front, but you do not have to be facing your partner to fondle them. Try something different. Stand behind her and with your front pressed against her back, massage them gently letting your fingers gently caress her taut peaks. From this angle, you have free roam over the entire front of her body. Along the lines of hitting that sweet spot on the breast, when it comes to putting them in your mouth, you also need to exercise caution. The nipples are incredibly sensitive. Some women are able to handle a little more pressure than others. Make sure you know what she likes and does not like before thinking about a little nibble. There are few things that will ruin the mood quicker than pain.

The sixth zone on a woman are the **ears.** There are several nerve endings in the ears from the lobe to the cartilage. They are close to the neck making it easy to go back and forth between the two erogenous zones to really get her excited. The lobes are not quite as sensitive as the nipples, so a little nibble is not going to kill the mood. As a matter of fact, statistics show many women do enjoy having their lobes nibbled on. That combined with the breath being lightly breathed on their neck and ears only heightens the sensuality of this type of foreplay.

The last zone (not in terms of overall number but the last for this book) is the area behind the **knees.** It might sound a bit accessible, but there are several positions during sex and *before* sex that make that ultra sensitive area easy to get to. Before sex, have your woman lie on her back and give her a massage. While you work her thighs and calves, lightly rub that area behind her knees. Kiss them, lick them...any kind of light touch will be sure to drive your woman wild. Keep in mind that some women are ticklish, which is where the right amount of pressure comes in. Ensuring you do not go too lightly will keep her from giggling.

Pleasure spots for him:

The first of these erogenous zones might come as a surprise. It is the **lower lip**. It does not include the entire lip, however. There is a slope that can be found in between the outside of his lower lip and chin that is incredibly sensitive. That little curve is full of super sensitive nerve receptors. While making out with your man, suck the lower lip and pull it into your mouth. Then, utilize the tip of your tongue by stroking it up and down that little curve just below his lip. That move arouses that entire zone in such a sexually provoking manner that it will really get him excited. By keeping that lower lip of his in your mouth, the sensation is amplified. This motion will make him feel as though little electrical currents surge straight from his mouth down to his shaft.

The second zone is the **front of the neck**. When it comes to this area, we tend to lick or suck on the side of the neck near the ears. Another area we tend to focus on is the collarbone. Those might work just fine, but it is not an area full of those sensitive nerves. The major point of stimulation is the spot just beneath the Adam's apple. Medical professionals refer to it as the thyroid. It is a gland shaped like a butterfly that is a little more than halfway down the front of the neck. It is linked, quite closely, to the sex organs, so says Chinese medicine practitioners. To activate this zone, you will want to have him lie down on his back. It is best to have a pillow behind his head so that his neck is arched forward ever so slightly and that Adam's apple is exposed. Tease him just a little by brushing your lips against the lowest part of his throat. (known as the hollow) After that, use the flat part of your tongue and slide it upward until you reach the Adam's apple. Because the thyroid is directly beneath it, dip back down slightly. Massage the whole area using circular, wide motions with the tongue. Those circles ensure the entire thyroid is covered, which gives him the maximum amount of pleasure. By the time you are done with him, he will be incredibly hot and bothered.

The third zone might sound like it is more geared toward a woman. Surprisingly enough, a man's **nipples** could be even more sensitive than those of a woman. This is likely due to the fact men are not used to having their nipples be the center of sexual attention. Most men's nipples are like uncharted territory in that they are erogenous zones that have yet to be experimented with. Touching them will send pleasurable shock waves throughout his entire body. The best trick with the nipples is known as the *ice cream swirl*. While he lays on his back, you will lick slow circles around the outside of his nipple. Start at the areola and make slow circles moving inward until you reach the nipple. This is a very tantalizing move with the tongue. Once you reach the nipple, give it a little flick with the tip of your tongue and then nip it ever so gently. Building up pleasure in that manner is something that men truly love. If you'd like to up the ante a little, suck on an ice cube for a while before you start. The coldness of your tongue supercharges the nerve endings of the nipple.

Another zone that might come as a surprise is the dip just underneath his **ankle.** This point is found about halfway between the ankle bone and heel. The pressure point is about the size of your fingertip and it has some serious erogenous potential. Amazingly enough, it is another area directly linked to your man's sex organ. By pressing into it, energy is released and produces pleasurable feelings as a result. The best way to literally get your man to blow a gasket is to ride your man in reverse (this move is called the reverse cowgirl). When you feel him near climax, reach down and grab his ankles. Put a little bit of pulsating pressure on the ankle in time with his thrusts.

The next zone we are going to cover is the **perineum.** Many men tend to be a little shy when it comes to talking about this area, or guiding you to it. It is the patch of skin just behind his sac. Beneath that is the prostate gland which is an organ with quite a bit of orgasmic power. Rubbing that gently will bring him to the brink of climax rather quickly. Just before he prepares to enter you, take his sac into your hands and rub them lightly. While your hand is down there, press the knuckles gently against the perineum. While you two are getting down and dirty, keep rubbing and kneading. Just as he is about to climax, press your knuckles a little deeper. That move will lengthen and intensify his orgasm.

It may seem that the **shaft** does not need mentioning. However, there is one move in particular that will really set your man on fire. For this particular move, have your man lay down comfortably on his back. Sit between his legs (they should be outstretched) and face him. Take your thumb and index finger and make two tight rings around his shaft. One will be at the top while the other is in the middle. Slide your *rings* in opposing directions moving from the base to the head moving both hands simultaneously. There will be tantalizing friction, especially if things start off particularly slow and teasingly. Speed up only to slow down again to add to the sexual tension. Lubricant isn't required, but it will make this action much more pleasurable for him, so give it a try. Either way, he is going to love it.

Mentioning the shaft brings us to the next part of the penis and that is the **head.** There are more receptors for pleasure at the head than in any other part of the penis. It can be difficult to apply the right amount of pressure. The kind that brings him sexual bliss, not the kind that makes him want to keep your mouth permanently away from his package. There is a specific maneuver you can use called *the lipstick trick.* To accomplish this, you will have your man lie on his back, his stiff member pointing upward. Take hold of the base with your fingers to hold him steady. Make sure you aren't using a fist, just the fingers. Keep your lips closed yet relaxed as you brush them against the head. Rub it over your wet mouth in a motion mimicking the application of lipstick. This sensation can be heightened by opening your lips slightly and rubbing the head in between them. On occasion, take the entire head into your mouth, then return to just rubbing the head against your lips. He will love being able to watch as you tease him with your luscious lips.

You know the crease on the **testicles** that seems to act as a partition for the boys? That is known as the seam and is one of the erogenous zones we are going to cover in this book. Apparently, it has a lot more pleasure sensors than we originally thought. In order to get to those super sensitive places, you will need to once again take the initiative. This area is sensitive though, so tread lightly. Take his sac in one hand, then gently press your index finger and middle finger of the other hand into the top part of the crease. This will be closest to where the sac meets the base of the penis. Trace a line down with your fingers until you get to the bottom of the scrotum. While still massaging with one hand, slide your fingers back up to the top once more. Those movements are sure to get him really aroused.

The last zone we are going to talk about in this chapter is the **frenulum.** Known as the *F spot*, it is the area of flesh that sits just under the crown of the penis and is where the shaft meets the head. It does not get much for attention, perhaps because it is not very noticeable, especially when the penis is fully erect. In order to excite him with this *F spot*, you will take the base of his penis in one hand and lick slow circles around the crown. Every time you circle back around to that frenulum, flick your tongue quickly over it a couple of times, then go back to licking circles around the crown. All the while, you will continue to work your hand up and down the shaft. This maneuver is sure to give him a mind-blowing orgasm.

Chapter 10: Final Thoughts

When it comes to sex, there are literally hundreds if not thousands of ways to please your partner. In conclusion, we will leave you with a few tips for each sex for you to keep in mind when pleasing your partner.

With men, remember that they want to feel desired too. Due to standards in society, women are often the objects of desire and men are considered the owners of desire. Sex is something we make happen which means it is something we can make exciting, fresh and new. A good way to make your man feel like he is the most desirable man alive is to just grab him. Yeah, we mean *there*. It is a great way to initiate sex and it makes your man feel wanted and desired. Morning sex is also a great way to start off the day. He will have a spring in his step and will be smiling all the way to work.

Where men want to feel, desired and love the idea of their partner pursuing them every once in a while, women often feel the same. It may sound strange because as we stated a moment ago, women are the object of desire. However nice it may be to have an attractive person take notice, it is far more desirable for the partner to take note of how beautiful their woman is. Tell her and show her regularly. Between work, children and household duties, women can sometimes find it difficult to feel sexy. Holding her hand in public, giving her a kiss on the cheek or even just telling her how beautiful she is are great ways of keeping your woman's confidence levels high. It also triggers those thoughts in her mind and will keep her revved up and ready to go.

You can also try to abstain from sex for a period of time. This is a great way to build some serious sexual tension. Holding off for a few days while in the interim touching and teasing each other will make for a truly orgasmic experience when the two of you do have sex. Do not forget the foreplay, though. Even though you have been building that sexual tension for the past couple of days, you still want to include foreplay. A good thing to remember is to include that pre sex game 99.9% of the time. The occasional quickie is obviously the exception to that rule.

Communicate with one another and provide direction. Remember that your partner does not have the same parts you do. They cannot see inside your head and do not really understand your likes and dislikes. If something does not feel good, tell them. Likewise, if something feels *really* good, make sure they know that too. Keep things as positive as you can when giving direction. You do not want it to sound rude or make your partner feel inadequate. That is a mood killer.

Earlier, we talked about role play, but did you know you can play games with your partner while naked? There are so many variations for you to choose from. Naked twister, naked charades, strip poker...the list goes on and on. You can take any game and turn it into sexy time just by removing an article of clothing every now and then. If you choose to play naked charades, try acting out the things you would like to do to your partner. Along the lines of games, you can also try a Simon Says or Do as I do. Each of you can take turns being in charge of the game. Start by touching yourself and have your partner mimic your movements. It is a super fun way to tease and tantalize.

We have discussed the occasional quickie and there is nothing a man likes more than a quick, unexpected session of naked fun. As a woman, you can learn to enjoy the occasional quickie. In the morning, get up a few minutes before him and prepare yourself. Do whatever you usually do when you stimulate yourself, only stop before you have an orgasm. Then, go out and wake your man up for some really hot impromptu sex. He will love it and so will you!

Earlier in this book, we discussed erogenous zones. There are many more than those we covered so take some time and really explore your partner's body. Find the zone that really gets them going but do not stop once you have found a new one. Continue to explore on a regular basis. It is all part of the fun of foreplay and having sex.

Focus on your partner. It is really easy to get distracted by everything we have going on in life from work and bills to children and family. Believe it or not, your partner will be able to tell that you are distracted. Clear your mind of anything and everything *not* related to sex. Have fun. You do not get nearly as many moments to enjoy one another as you should. When the opportunity does arise, you are going to want to take full advantage of it.

Keep things spicy. Find new places to have sex. Obviously you need to be careful of public places as that is against the law. There are probably unchartered territories in your house. You can try the kitchen counter, the table, the bathroom sink. Up against the wall or bedroom door is always fun.

From new places to new positions, it is always fun to explore new horizons. In addition to Tantra, you can look into the art of Kama Sutra. Like Tantra, it has been around for ages and it is an amazing method to try, especially if you and your partner shy away from things like role play, exhibitionism, swinging or threesomes. Tantra and Kama Sutra are ways for you and your partner to explore one another and realize that special, ultra deep connection that makes relationships stronger and healthier. When we are talking about broadening your sexual horizons, it just means to try something you may not think you will like. After all, you never know until you give it a try. Push your sexual limits and have a great time doing it!

Conclusion

Thank you again for purchasing this book!

I hope this book was able to help you to learn the true meaning of BDSM, its basics, and its benefits.

The next step is to apply these tips and strategies to bring your sex life and your relationship to exhilarating heights.

Lastly, remember that sex is meant to be an extraordinary experience, so don't be afraid of exploring activities and sensations that are beyond the ordinary. Each of us has our own fetishes and fantasies. Are you brave enough to live out yours?

Finally, if you enjoyed this book, then I'd like to ask you for a favor, would you be kind enough to leave a review for this book on Amazon? It'd be greatly appreciated!

Thank you and good luck!

BONUS: Preview of our fiction book Taming the Tigress: A Journey To Submission

Chapter 1: Caged

Punishment

I awoke in pitch blackness. I was all alone. I waited for it to come... the dread, the panic. It didn't. At first, I thought that the cold had numbed me, body and soul. But then I remembered. And I felt the stirrings of excitement in my gut, the involuntary clench of my cunt, triggered by the remembrance of the night before.

Was it really last night that he came here? Or was it the night before that? I could scarcely remember.

In the dungeon, there were neither days nor nights. Only darkness bleeding into further darkness. I counted my days not by the mornings or the evenings. No, the Master was my universe, my rising and my setting sun. My days began with his touch. And my days died each time he left. His touch... oh I tried to remember it. I shivered in the cold and tried to recall the warmth of his hands encircling my ankles, travelling up my legs, my thighs, tracing the triangle of my pubic hair. He took his sweet time knowing fully well how he was torturing me. At this memory, lust spread like wildfire all over my body. I remembered everything with stunning precision although the occasions when he would actually touch me seemed so rare compared to the moments I spent alone in the dungeon.

I felt the ache in my stretched muscles. In the dungeon, every single inch of my body was alive with pain. Yet every fiber of my being tingled with excitement. My hands were cuffed and tied to a high pole. My legs were spread wide apart. My toes were barely touching the cold stone floor. Time trundled at a snail's pace and I spent the hours wavering between consciousness and unconsciousness, teetering between sanity and madness. I would strain my ears listening to the sounds of his footsteps, hoping he would come. There were times when I could've sworn I heard his footsteps. They were heavy, leisurely, torturous... Yet I would hear the sound stop just outside the door. I would hear the rasping sound of his breathing, sense the heat of his body from the other side. At those times, I would be tempted to call out his name, to beg him to come to me. But then I'd remember what the Master had said to me: "Not a sound, *mon chaton.*"

Ah yes, he called me his kitten. I was his pet. His strokes were always gentle. Until I misbehaved. Then he brought me to the dungeon.

Once, I dared myself to call him. Just once. Just so I could feel him near me again. When I first opened my mouth, it was as if my tongue had been severed. I tried to scream out his name but it came out as a dry croak. My throat was parched. I hadn't drunk anything in days.

He saw me, of course. I had no idea how many hours he spent looking at me from the monitor in his bedroom.

He came for me then. My Master, my Savior. A weak yellow light tiptoed into the room and I felt the familiar damp sensation spreading between my thighs. The Master carried a gas lamp in one hand and a bucket of water in the other.

He let me drink tiny sips from his open palms. I licked his palms clean, wasting not a single drop. I kept licking his palms, flicking my tongue against his hard flesh. He flipped his hand and I licked the back of it, lovingly, eagerly; perhaps a bit too eagerly because he pulled it suddenly away from me.

I looked into his eyes beseechingly. *Please, take me.* I thought, though I dared not speak the words out loud. *Please.*

He shook his head slowly. Then he walked away, leaving me sobbing in the dark. I knew then that that was my punishment for attempting to speak.

Reward

I knew that my obedience would not be for nothing. I heard his footsteps. They were quick, decisive, urgent.

The Master wanted me and he wanted me then and there.

The door swung open and I kept my gaze downward, not daring to ruin things by being too presumptuous. His breathing was heavy and I saw the bulk of his cock straining rebelliously against the fabric of his trousers. I knew my obedience had turned him on. Inside, I rejoiced. I knew I did well. I behaved and stayed put and waited for him in that dungeon. It was time for my reward.

He produced the key from his pocket and yet despite his obvious urgency, he unlocked the cuffs and untied the ropes slowly. My knees were so weak and my muscles were extremely exhausted that I fell towards him.

The Master caught me in his arms. His breath was hot in my ear as he whispered: "Lie down, Katharine."

I lay down and the coldness of the stone was cruel. It didn't matter.

"Good, my pet." he said. "Now, keep your hands on your sides."

So I did. My legs were splayed, ready to receive him. My palms flat on the floor.

The Master knelt in front of me, unzipped his trousers and freed his furious flesh.

He grabbed my ankles and raised my legs so they were pointing toward the ceiling. Then he pushed them down towards me so that my feet were on either side of my head. I became extremely aware of how exposed I was to him.

Without warning, he impaled me with a single penetrating fuck. He pierced me, flesh and soul. I screamed with pleasure and gratitude.

He moved in and out of me and with each filling thrust, his balls slapped hard against my cunt. My moist cunt involuntarily convulsed around his rigid cock and my love liquid poured generously around him.

He gasped.

I looked up to see his handsome leonine face. It was contorted in ecstasy. For a brief moment, just before he shuddered and released his hot spunk into me, I caught a glimpse of a side of him that I rarely saw.

I always wished I could freeze time, capture that image of him, and hold it forever. But right now, I am his slave. He is my Master.

How did I get here?

I *wanted* to be here, had begged to be here. I wanted to surrender my life into his hands.

Chapter 2: The Tigress

How did I get here?

It all started with an awkward incident at the ladies' room.

"The Tigress was at it again this morning." said the whiny voice that trickled from the bathroom stall. "I find it really hard to concentrate on my work when she's like literally breathing down my neck."

Laughter oozed from the other stall. "Looks like someone needs to get laid."

My first reaction was fury. Who the fuck do these bitches think they are? They work for *me*. Then I realized how pathetic that sounded. Me, bullied by my own employees. I didn't even know what their names were or what departments they're from.

The Tigress. That's what they called me. I used to think that it was a fond nickname, owing to my fierceness and my success. Until I realized that it wasn't.

I waited for the women to come out. When they did, I looked at their pale faces and said: "You're fired. Both of you."

Then I left, feeling terrible over my extreme immaturity.

"They *love* working for you." Joan, my secretary, who is also coincidentally my only friend at the office, told me. "But they also hate working for you. If that makes any sense..."

It did make sense. I was too uptight. My ill temper was contagious. Somehow, with my controlling attitude, I created a hostile work environment for my employees.

I decided to take the afternoon off and asked Joan to cancel my next two appointments.

"How did the delivery go?" I picked up my purse, ready to leave.

I was talking about the anonymous client who ordered chartreuse silk dresses by the bulk. Here's the catch: Through the past year, it was always several pieces of the exact same design, color, and size. It was weird. The money, though, was always paid up front. In fact, I owed the expansion of my little dress shop partly to that client's patronage. So I figured, if she wanted to use that single design as some sort of disposable daily uniform, then so be it.

That's not to say that I hadn't been curious. In fact, I used to be the one who personally delivered the dresses to the mansion. It was always received by different maids whose bland faces betrayed nothing. I knew that the mansion was owned by Louis Archambault as in Archambault Pharmaceuticals. But as far as I knew, there was no Mrs. Archambault.

I tried Googling him, of course. Apparently, he's a very private person. He was handsome, disturbingly so; a tall man with piercing eyes. In his photos, his lips were curled to form a curt half-smile... a cold, almost cruel curve. But I had a feeling that they could be warm and tender when he wanted them to be.
I even went so far as to send him a thank you gift: a dress of a different design. Then I got flowers and a formal thank you note, no doubt written by his secretary. After a while, I just gave up trying to find out who the gowns were for. For all I knew, they were for him. Still, for some ridiculous reason, I kept his picture in one of my folders. I looked at it from time to time.

"They're still here." Joan's voice punctured my thoughts.

"What?"

"The gowns are still here. Winona was supposed to deliver them."

"Well, why didn't she?" I asked, starting to get irritated.

"Um, you just fired her…"

"Shit."

#

Before I could even bother to introduce myself, the new maid ushered me into the house while the other unloaded the boxes from my car. It was my first time to see the mansion's interior. It was palatial.

"You're late." she scolded.

"Oh." I said. "I know. I'm so--"

"Shush!" She cut me off, harshly. "He'll be here soon. Let's get you ready."

I hardly paid attention to what she said after that. I let her drag me up the stairs.

He'll be here soon… That was all I could think about. *Him!*

So I played along, not thinking about the consequences.

Until then, it didn't really occur to me how badly I wanted to meet him. One peek, I told myself. And then I'll come clean.

When she slipped me into one of the silk dresses, I realized that it was my size.

So, I thought. *Mr. Archambault likes his escorts in my green dresses.* And the maid mistook me for one of them. I wasn't exactly sure how I felt about that.

I was led into his office.

And there he was in all his dominant glory.

"Sit." he said sharply.

I found myself automatically dropping into a chair.

"Not there." He said again. He pressed his hand on his desk. "Here."

There was a magnetism in his voice that I couldn't resist. Without peeling my gaze from his lion-like face and without understanding myself, I sat on the edge of the table.

When his fingers dug into my shoulders, I felt the energy from his touch. The current traveled all the way from my shoulders to my clit. I pressed my legs together. I was starting to get wet. He lifted my skirt and pried my legs open with one swift gesture. Blood rushed to my face as I realized that he was smiling at the swiftly spreading puddle of pussy juice on my panties.

I opened my mouth but my indignant protest came out as a gasp.

He had entered me with his fingers, a heavenly assault.

Then, he withdrew his hand up to his lips to taste me.

"It's nice to finally meet you, Ms. Mallory."

He flashed me his cold, cruel half-grin and for a fleeting moment, I felt fear.

Instinctively, I got to my feet and raised my hand to slap him. But he caught it and in one deft movement, he turned me over so that I was leaning facedown onto the table.

He pulled down my panties. I felt his erection pressing against my ass. I trembled with anticipation. I expected him to enter me roughly from behind.

Slap!

The ruler landed on my bum, causing the flesh to sting.

Then he ran his palm soothingly over my smarting butt cheeks.

"I do not tolerate tardiness." he said.

Slap!

The ruler came down, harder this time.

Was he *punishing* me?

I ought to have stopped him. I ought to have run away. I ought to have done a lot of things.

But I stayed.

Slap!

Tears stung my eyes.

"*Never* raise your hand against me!" he said roughly into my ear.

I heard the silk ripping away beneath his hands. My body flooded with proportionate amounts of lust and fear.

"Beautiful." he sighed. "You are a blank canvass."

But he didn't fuck me like I hoped he would.

Instead, I listened to his breath waxing and waning as he masturbated.

I tried to face him but he held my head down, my cheeks pressed hard against the table.

"Stay down." he ordered. "You are no lioness. You are my little kitten. That's all you are, *mon chaton.*"

"Yes." I murmured, tears stinging my eyes. "Yes."

I felt him shudder. And a deluge of hot semen rained down my back and trickled down my still burning bum.

He walked away, leaving me there, bent over, covered in his jizz, my cunt still wet and aching for him.

I cried. At that moment, I knew. He broke me. And I've never felt more alive.

Check out rest of the book for FREE! All you have to do is to join our list. Look at Amazon for More Sex More Fun Book Club!

Made in the USA
Middletown, DE
06 October 2022

12141735R00036